I0441998

Detox Diet:
Eating Well For A Life Of Pure Energy, Shape And Health.

Copyright © 2015, Remy Roulier

TABLE OF CONTENTS

I- THE POWER TO RECOVER TODAY ALL YOUR ENERGY, SHAPE AND HEALTH

The core principles (4 powers and 4 poisons) you are about to discover will allow you to create an extraordinary energy, shape and health, by making a deep and complete analysis of every kind of food and beverage that goes in your stomach every day.

They are about to detoxify yourself completely and you are going to learn something essential: **how to eat well**.

And yet, this so simple thing has become so difficult to learn.

You want to know why?

This is mainly due to the endless lies the food industry wants you to believe, often for their own economic interests and absolutely not for your health.

Maybe you already use some of the principles you are going to learn here.

This program is designed to maximize the potential of your body and mind, in order to enjoy exceptional health.

Best of all, these principles will not require you more time; they are simple, fast and fun!

II- THE POWER OF WATER AND LIVING FOODS

Water is a major component of all living matter. This is the main component of the human body.

Water represents 76% of your brain, 90% of your lungs, 84% of your blood and 98% of your blood plasma.

The vital processes such as digestion, blood circulation and excretion are impossible without water.

Water carries nutrients to all vital organs, it plays an essential role in maintaining the body at the right temperature and contributes to its growth and regeneration.

Water is the second most important element for your health after oxygen, without which you would die within minutes.

An adult can live for several weeks without food, but not more than ten days without water.

Your body can not afford to lose more than 10% of its water to stay alive.

II.1- The Experience Of Dr Ferrydoon Batmanghelidj

Dr. Batmanghelidj was a political prisoner in Iran. He was placed in solitary confinement during his detention. He decided not to consume food during this period because he believed that without exercise or without movement, food would become toxic for his body.

Thus, during seven days, he ate almost nothing and drank only water. He was amazed to note that water completely relieved pain associated with hunger.

After this period of isolation, he was transferred to the main wing of the prison where were 300 other prisoners.

One night, some prisoners brought him a man feeling terrible pain. The guards refused to take him to the hospital, and Dr. Batmanghelidj was his last hope.

Because he didn't have any drugs to give to the prisoner, Dr. Batmanghelidj made him drink two glasses of water. In the minutes that followed, the man started to feel much better and his pain decreased consistently.

Dr. Batmanghelidj asked for two glasses of water every three hours during the four months they spent in the same block. He was astonished by the result: the man was suffering from a stomach ulcer and yet the water relieved his pain.

After this promising experience, Dr. Batmanghelidj developed a passion for water used as a medicine, and devoted the rest of his time in prison to carry out scientific research on the effects of water. During the two years and seven months of his incarceration, he healed about 3,000 other similar cases.

He finally settled in the United States, where the results of his research were published in the Journal of Clinical Gastroentrology. Later, he was hired by the University of Pennsylvania to continue his research. Its first conclusions show that medicine has given many names to the various stages of dehydration, and that water can play an important role not only to maintain health, but also to cure this disease.

Dr. Batmanghelidj died in November 2004. His work continues to influence many people, but he is deeply missed for his multiple skills as a researcher, pioneer, husband and father.

The following pages contain a summary of his work.

II.2- The Causes Of Dehydration

Our current activities make us lose an average of 2.5 liters per day. This quantity is usually replaced by what we drink and the food we eat.

But exercise, sweat, diarrhea, fever or altitude can dramatically increase our fluid intake needs.

Exercise and sweat are the most common causes of dehydration. Only a slight dehydration is enough to decrease coordination, create fatigue and impair judgment. It is through breathing, sweating, urination and defecation that liquids leave our body. This phenomenon will be more or less fast depending on the level of activity, ambient humidity, air temperature and altitude.

II.3- The Symptoms Of Dehydration

A dry mouth is the last external sign of dehydration. In addition, the perception of thirst decreases with age.

If you are thirsty, it means that your cells are already dehydrated.

A **severely** dehydrated body produces orange or dark urine.

A **slightly** dehydrated body produces yellow urine.

A **properly** hydrated body produces colorless urine.

Some of the side effects of dehydration are: stress, headaches, back pain, allergies, weight gain, asthma, hypertension and Alzheimer's disease.

ALCOHOL AND CAFFEINE KILL YOU SLOWLY

Alcohol stops the reverse osmosis process, which allows water to penetrate into the cells.

Caffeine stimulates the kidneys to excrete more water than that contained initially in the caffeinated drink. It also inhibits the enzymes that ensure the proper functioning of the memory.

II.4- What Quantity Of Water Should You Drink Daily?

You should drink daily half of your body weight in ounces.

For example, if your weight is 200 pounds, you should drink 100 ounces of water every day.

Ideally, you should never stay more than 15 to 20 minutes without taking a sip of water.

You should start to drink water in the morning before getting out of bed This is indeed the time when you are the most toxic and dehydrated.

You should always drink water before eating to ease digestion.

****
DRINK HALF OF YOUR WEIGHT IN OZ EVERY DAY!
If you weigh 200 pounds, you should drink 100 ounces
****

II.5- Percentage Of Water In Common Foods

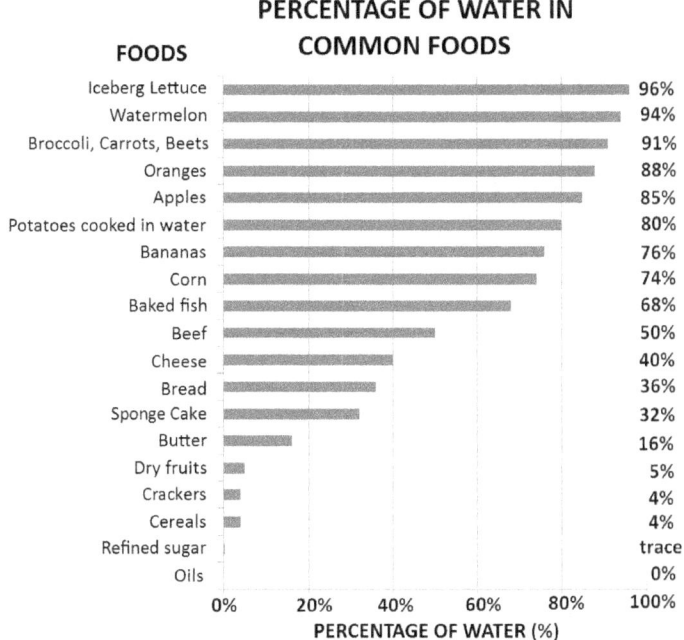

PERCENTAGE OF WATER IN COMMON FOODS

FOODS	PERCENTAGE OF WATER (%)
Iceberg Lettuce	96%
Watermelon	94%
Broccoli, Carrots, Beets	91%
Oranges	88%
Apples	85%
Potatoes cooked in water	80%
Bananas	76%
Corn	74%
Baked fish	68%
Beef	50%
Cheese	40%
Bread	36%
Sponge Cake	32%
Butter	16%
Dry fruits	5%
Crackers	4%
Cereals	4%
Refined sugar	trace
Oils	0%

II.6- Test Yourself: How Much Water And Living Foods Do You Consume?

1- Write down everything that went through your mouth in the last 24 hours:

_____

_____

_____

_____

_____

_____

_____

_____

_____

_____

_____

_____

_____

_____

DIET OF A SINGLE MAN: 36 HOURS OF GASTRONOMY

DIET OF ONE HUMAN FOOD 36 HOURS

1 Milky Way
1 Ground beef pizza
1 Big Mac
1 Roasted duck
3 cold cereal bowls with skim milk
3 Pears
3 Melons
1 Pasta Dish
1 Popcorn Pack like in a cinema
2 Madeleines
10 Sparkling beverages
1 Ham sandwich

2- Look at the list of everything that went through your mouth over the past 24 hours. What percentage of your diet consists of foods rich in water?

_____
_____
_____
_____
_____
_____
_____
_____
_____
_____
_____
_____
_____
_____

****
EVERY TIME YOU ARE ABOUT TO EAT SOMETHING, ASK
YOURSELF THE QUESTION:
"IS THIS FOOD GOING TO PURIFY ME...OR CLOG MY
BODY?"
****

3- Name some water-rich foods that you enjoy:

_____

_____

_____

_____

_____

_____

_____

_____

_____

_____

_____

_____

_____

_____

_____

(If you need inspiration, feel free to use the histogram of the chapter II.5).

II.7- Summary

At least 70% of your diet should consist of foods rich in water.

This is what allows your body to self-purify. If you consume less than 70% of water-rich foods, you clog your body, instead of purifying it.

The typical diet in the Americas, Europe, Asia, Australia, etc., is only made of 15% of water-rich foods. In other words: it is <u>suicide</u>!

'Water is the mother of the vine, the nurse and fountain of fecundity, the adorner and refresher of the world.'
Charles Mackay, the Dionysia

III- THE POWER OF ESSENTIAL OILS

This chapter deals with the power of fats. We live in a society where the media constantly bombard us with messages about products designed to remove all fats from our diet.

There is an endless list of "light" products: sweet or salted biscuits, cakes or breads, pasta, salad dressings, crisps or cereal bars.

However, few people realize that completely removing fats from our diet is the worst thing to do!

In reality, fats are very important in our diet and our health; all the secret lies in knowing what are the good fats and what are the fats that can kill.

Essential fatty acids are healthy or cleansing fats: every cell in our body needs to function, especially our brain that is made of 60% of fat content.

These good fats are essential fatty acids: Omega-3 and Omega-6. Your body needs them to survive. Without them, the lipid bilayer surrounding your cells starts to disintegrate.

III.1- 12 Reasons Why Essential Fatty Acids Are Important For A Healthy Life

1- They contribute to many vital functions in cells, tissues and organs. They increase the oxidation and basal metabolism. The energy and strength increase and the recovery time decreases.

2- Skin Care: In addition to making the skin soft and silky, they help reduce acne, psoriasis and eczema.

3- Digestion: they help prevent intestinal porosity that can cause allergies, inflammation and autoimmune problems.

4- In the cardiovascular system, they are required to transport cholesterol, short triglycerides, reduce platelet adhesion and lower blood pressure.

5- They improve mood, alleviate depression and improve our ability to handle stress. High stress levels cause hypertension, fluid retention, inflammation and blood clots.

6- It regulates heartbeat and prevents abnormal heart rhythms (arrhythmia) that can lead to a heart attack.

7- Overweight people and animals have a direct benefit because their kidneys drain water in excess.

8- In the immune system, they protect the integrity of the DNA. They are not a treatment for people or animals with cancer, but they are very beneficial. Greases are a nutritional adjuvant for the immune and cardiovascular systems.

9- It decreases inflammation among people who suffer from osteoarthritis and rheumatoid arthritis.

10- They participate in the transport of minerals in the body.

11- The brain cannot function without them.

12- Research has shown that the unborn child draws in the body of his mother substantial amounts of essential fatty acids to develop his brain.

III.2- The Best Sources Of Essential Oils

1- Twinlab Krill Oil

This product from the sea offers all the benefits of Omega-3 and biologically active compounds such as EPA and DHA. It contains natural antioxidants (Vitamins A and E, Astaxanthin-a, carotenoids and flavonoids). Krill oil is in a phospholipid form, which allows the body to assimilate it easily.

The krill (like the shrimp) is a renewable species that is positioned in a lower level in the food chain. This is why it remains almost unaffected by industrial toxins that contaminate most fishes.

It can be consumed as it is, and should not be subjected to high temperatures during the transformation. Studies proved that taking only 300mg a day already starts to provide positive results.

Twinlab's Krill Oil (Krill Essentials ™) is on sale in most natural and/or vitamins food stores. Each capsule contains 72mg of Omega-3.

2- Udo's Choice Oil Blend

Udo's Choice Ultimate Oil Blend is a special blend of essential oils, unrefined. It contains linseed oil, fresh sesame and sunflower from organically certified plantations oil, and wheat germ, rice and oats oils.

This oil blend is rich in lecithin (the component of healthy cell membranes), medium chain triglycerides (MCTs are easy to digest and to assimilate and are used as an energy source) and vitamin E to improve product life and to protect the body from free radicals.

Udo's Choice Oil is natural, unrefined and contains a perfectly balanced blend of essential fatty Omega 3 acids (alpha-linoleic acid) and Omega-6 acids (linoleic). These fatty acids are essential for survival, but they cannot be created by the body and must come from food.

Studies have shown that the traditional occidental diet doesn't contain enough Omega-3. However, too much Omega-3 and Omega-6 can cause some malfunctions.

Udo's Choice Oil Blend is designed to bring together in a single product the two fatty acids in the right quantities: a ratio of two Omega-3 for one Omega-6.

The best way to absorb this oil is to drink a glass or pour it over your salad or other food once you cooked them. Udo's Oil should never be heated and must be kept in the refrigerator.

****

RECOMMENDED QUANTITY: TAKE ONE SOUP SPOON FOR EVERY 55 POUNDS OF BODY WEIGHT EVERY DAY. FOR EXAMPLE, IF YOU WEIGH 165 POUNDS, YOU MAY TAKE 3 SOUP SPOONS PER DAY.

****

IV- THE POWER OF ALKALINITY: GO GREEN!

When our body is imbalanced and we lack energy, we face a whole series of problems, such as stress, fatigue, depression and disease.

To stay healthy, it is essential to have a balanced blood chemical composition and to have an adequate ratio of acid and alkaline foods in your diet. In fact, an excess of acidity in tissues causes different types of health status, from lethargy and fatigue, to obesity or much more serious health problems.

One of the main priorities of our body is to make sure that the alkalinity level always remains high enough to ensure cellular life. Control mechanisms such as breathing, blood circulation, digestion and hormone production ensure the body to have a balanced pH by eliminating the acid residues contained in the tissues. If the pH becomes too acid or too alkaline, the cells are poisoned by their own toxic wastes, and they die.

THE pH SCALE:

This scale measures the acidity or alkalinity level of a substance. pH stands for "potential Hydrogen". Acids have a pH below 7, and alkali have a pH greater than 7. A substance with a pH of 7 is neutral: neither acidic nor alkaline.

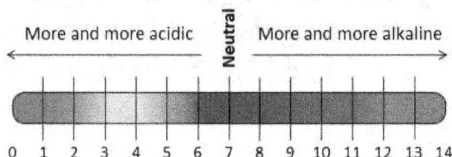

The various tissues of the body must maintain a different pH to nourish life.

Blood and most tissues must remain slightly alkaline, while the urine, saliva and digestive system should be slightly acidic.

In fact, the blood can tolerate only slight fluctuations in pH to stay healthy.

Yet the most important thing is the alkali reserve of the body (composed of elements such as baking soda) that is stored to be able to neutralize, if necessary, an excess of acid in the body. If the body becomes too acidic or depletes its alkali reserves, the cells will start to weaken and to divide, and the body functions will be compromised.

IV.1- Consequences Of An Unbalanced/Hyper Acidic pH

1- If you are overweight, you probably do not have a problem of 'fat', but a problem of acidity! The excess of acidity in the body, or acidosis, has two consequences: first, it may make the body produce more insulin and thus to store more fat. Then the cells under constant pressure to produce more insulin will split.

2- Too much acidity reduces affinity of hemoglobin for oxygen in your blood. When the oxygen supply to the cells decreases, all the body functions are in danger.

3- The degradation of the cell wall and membrane by free radicals is accelerated. This causes premature aging, vision and memory problems, wrinkles, age spots, hormonal disorders, etc.

4- When the blood plasma becomes more acidic, it acts as a chemical irritant that attacks and slowly devours the soft muscle tissue on the inner wall of arteries and veins, weakening their structural composition and causing uneven tension.

5- It becomes more difficult to control high blood pressure due to heart overwork.

6- Acidosis disrupts the normal metabolism of fatty acids and lipids, which causes neurological problems and hormonal imbalances in the endocrine system, which may increase the probability of disorders and urinary tract infections.

7- The acidity increases the probability of cells mutations.

8- Normal electrolytic activity is affected by a hyper acidic environment.

9- Access of the body to its energy reserves decreases because the normal cellular and body metabolism is inhibited.

10- An acidic pH allows the cholesterol to ally with heavy metals and other cellular debris, and thus accelerates the development of plaques in the vascular network.

IV.2- Have Fun And Make It Simple

1- Put lemon in the water you drink throughout the day.

2- Use lemon and a bit of good salt (Himalayan salt or Celtic sea salt) in the vinaigrette. Or make your own vinaigrette with recipes from your local natural store (linseed oil, lemon juice, Bragg® Liquid Aminos, pepper and garlic make a great combination!)

3- Replace white bread and wheat pizza dough with sprouted wheat bread and pizzas.

4. Diversify textures: tortilla chips with fresh guacamole, crisp vegetables with fresh hummus (mashed chickpeas), pita bread or sprouted wheat tortillas with avocado, dried tomatoes (which add a lot of flavor) with a little bit of soy cheese with spices, almond cream on a sprouted wheat toast, cream of broccoli with crunchy vegetables, etc.

5. Always have a fresh salad in the fridge, ready to use.

6. Use spices: Bragg® Liquid Aminos, Spice Hunter spices (or any spices from a natural food store), fresh herbs, Celtic sea salt, etc.

7- Drink one to four ounces of wheatgrass daily. Start with less and gradually increase the amount. You will find wheat grass in natural food stores or in juice bars.

8- A fresh smoothie or vegetable juice can soothe your sweet tooth, especially when the weather is hot.

Test new blends of flavors and textures,

and above all: have fun!
You can also find many books full of great recipes in
natural food stores.

IV.3- Why Is Wheatgrass So Precious?

In addition to chlorophyll, wheat grass provides the following nutrients to the body:

1- Vitamins: Wheatgrass has a high content of:

- Vitamin A (bone growth, sight and reproduction)
- Vitamin B (development of the brain and body, adrenal glands, nervous and digestive systems)
- Vitamin C (preservation of skin health, teeth, gums, eyes, muscles and joints)
- Vitamin E (helps the heart and reproductive system, vitamin E is more readily absorbed by the body than synthetic vitamins)

2- Minerals: 92 of the 102 existing minerals in the soil are absorbed by wheatgrass, including:

- Calcium (strengthens bones and teeth, regulates heart rate and helps to balance the blood pH)
- Iron (contributes to the formation of red blood cells and carries oxygen towards the cells)
- Sodium (digestion, elimination and regulation of body fluids)
- Potassium (body balance, muscle tone, firm skin)
- Magnesium (muscle function and elimination)

3- Amino Acids: Wheatgrass contains 17 amino acids, including the 8 essential amino acids (which constitute the proteins in the body). These are the 8 amino acids that our body cannot manufacture and must be synthesized from the food we eat.

4- <u>Enzymes:</u> Wheatgrass contains many enzymes and stimulates the production by the body of its own enzymes.

5-Wheatgrass <u>stimulates peristaltic activity and strengthens the functioning of the thyroid</u>.

V- THE POWER OF OPTIMAL NUTRITION

Although we are aware of what we eat, we do not always think about the meaning or purpose of this action.

To understand the importance of optimal nutrition, we must first understand the reason why we want to get there. Why trying to achieve an optimal nutrition? What will happen if we do not eat the right foods, or if we do not absorb the proper nutrients?

To understand the basics of good nutrition, we should first answer some basic questions.

V.1- Why Do We Eat?

1- To energize us

Food is a great asset when we have to manage our emotions and build energy reserves for our body. Healthy nutrients consumption can help you express what you feel and bring out a positive and radiant state of mind.

In addition, the right foods help your body to work perfectly and give you the energy you need to work, to take care of your family, to go to the gym, etc.

On the contrary, if you eat poorly, you lose all energy and you will feel lethargic, mentally and physically.

2- To grow and develop

What we eat should help us to regulate and maintain bodily functions. We carefully plan our food needs for the different stages of growth, to ensure the proper development of the body.

3- To purify us and cleanse us

We want to start every day with a clean slate, feeling fresh and revitalized. Our bodies need to be clean to function effectively and without hindrance. We must also absorb cleansing foods to take care of our appearance and maintain our skin.

4- To prevent and fight against disease

To fight against disease, we must offer our bodies a healthy ground.
Food helps us provide a solid base for a strong inner environment. In addition, food comfort us and help us to treat a variety of ailments, from little pain to killer diseases.

5- To feed our external beauty

Nutrients facilitate basic bodily functions, but they also contribute to our physical appearance. A poor diet can make us tired or sallow, while a healthy diet can shine our hair and promote our skin's health.

6- To socialize and have fun

Eating allows us to feed the human being inside us, and brings us closer to others in different social occasions. We learn to share, to celebrate, to love through food; we use it to comfort or to show our compassion.

However, we must be aware of its negative influences and know how to avoid them, so that eating remains a pleasure.

V.2- What Do We Give To Our Body?

Here are the seven food components:

Carbohydrates, proteins, fats, vitamins, minerals, water and fibers.

1- Fats (saturated, monounsaturated, polyunsaturated)

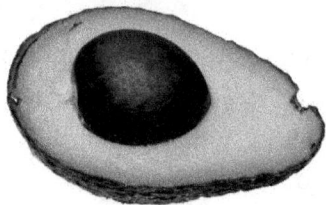

Fats are a concentrated of energy; they contribute to the absorption of fat soluble vitamins; they insulate the body; they protect the organs.

Fatty acids, glycerol, cholesterol: fats from foods provide essential fatty acids that the body cannot manufacture.

2- Carbohydrates (sugars, fibers, starches)

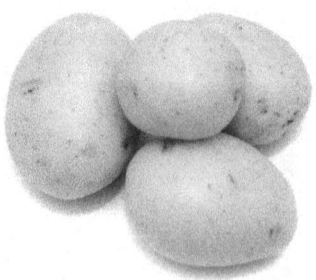

Most carbohydrates, which are the main fuel for the body, are metabolized to glucose.

Glucose is the main source of energy for the cells. Excess of carbohydrates is converted to glycogen which is stored in the liver and muscles.

3- Proteins (animal, plant)

Proteins are the building blocks of the cells, they are also known as amino acids (20 in total, 10 essential).

They preserve the cells of the muscles, tendons and ligaments.

The liver converts amino acids into a form of carbohydrate when the glycogen stock is almost depleted.

4- Water, Vitamins, Minerals

These components are also required to maintain the bodily functions.

****

The daily goal is to eat foods that will best contribute to these functions.
But the goal here is not only to provide you with this knowledge, but to nourish your body and mind of this information that will make you stronger and take you to a level of superior well-being.

V.3- The Seven Rules To Eat Healthy

1- Drink water before and after meals, never during.

Drink before the meal will fill your stomach and keep you from overeating. In addition, by refraining from drinking water, you can breathe properly, which will facilitate digestion.

Drink water 30 minutes before eating and do not drink water 10 (ideally 30) minutes before or after a meal.

2- Combine foods properly.

It is important to properly combine foods to digest the nutrients they contain. A bad combination of foods is burdening the digestive system. The consequences are, among others:

- Deferred Digestion. The food is not converted into nutrients, which does not allow us to take benefit from the amino acids, vitamins and minerals they contain.

- Harmful toxins. These poisons attach to our body cells and tissues, preventing the organs to remove them correctly.

- "Food Allergies". We often tend to confuse the discomfort that follows meals with food allergies, while it is simply the result of poor food combinations.

- More severe aches. A bad combination of food for an extended period can weaken the body and lead to more serious problems.

However, if we combine our food the good way, the digestive organs will continue to fulfill their normal function, and food can be properly digested. In addition, we will consume less energy to digest, which will allow us to absorb more nutrients that will give us energy.

THINK ABOUT THIS...

According to the American Association Food, here are the ideal portions:

1- A portion of pasta of the size of a tennis ball
2- A half portion of vegetables of the size of a bulb
3- A small baked potato of the size of a mouse

RUMINATE THAT:

Digestion is impaired by the consumption of condiments, vinegar, alcohol, tobacco, soft drinks, tea, coffee and cold drinks.

****

PRINCIPLES OF FOOD COMBINATIONS

(*Source: Food Combining Made Easy, Herbert Shelton, M.D.*)

Your diet should consist of 70% of alkaline foods, rich in water, and these foods can be combined only with a concentrated food (in order words, that does not contain a lot of water, such as meat, a baked potato or fish).

1. Always dissociate proteins and carbohydrates.
2. A green salad can always be combined with proteins, carbohydrates or lipids.
3. Always eat fruits separately, and don't mix them with any other kind of food.
4. Fats inhibit the digestion process of proteins. If you eat fats with proteins, you should also eat a mixed vegetables salad to counteract the inhibitory effect.
5. Never drink during or immediately after meals.

****

3- Be relaxed when you eat.

- Eliminate distractions, including television and the Internet.

- Stay calm. Meals should be a quiet moment to appreciate and fully enjoy the company of others and what you have in your plate.

- Everyone must be seated and at ease; prepare the table without forgetting anything.

- Chew slowly, and make small bites.

4- Eat reasonable amounts of food.

Among others, Americans have a completely distorted picture of portions. The portions served in restaurants are generally disproportionate: half of a portion would be widely enough. If you prepared too much food for dinner, keep what remains for lunch the next day.

Eat less ... To eat more.

After determining a healthy diet, you might also decide to reduce your calorie intake.

Dr. Roy Walford, a supporter of calorie restriction who participated in the Biosphere 2 project, recommends limiting your daily intake to live longer.

According to him, a diet low in fats and calories but rich in nutrients can make you live longer and increase your resistance to disease.

5- Eat organic.

Always eat food without pesticides, antibiotics or growth hormones. Products labeled "organic" have been approved by the USDA, which verifies that farms meet the standards adopted by the Government (including those aimed to promote renewable resources).

It was sometimes difficult to buy organic products a few years ago, but now we can find them everywhere. Even the small grocery store in the corner of the street is likely to have a shelf with natural products.

You may even have small supermarkets with natural, fresh and organic products close to you, or even organic markets.

6- The timing makes all the difference: eat small amounts every 3 hours.

7. Add supplements to your diet if necessary.

V.4- Food Combinations Table

This logical table below shows how a right combination of fresh and healthy food contributes to better digestion and more energy, while strengthening your body.

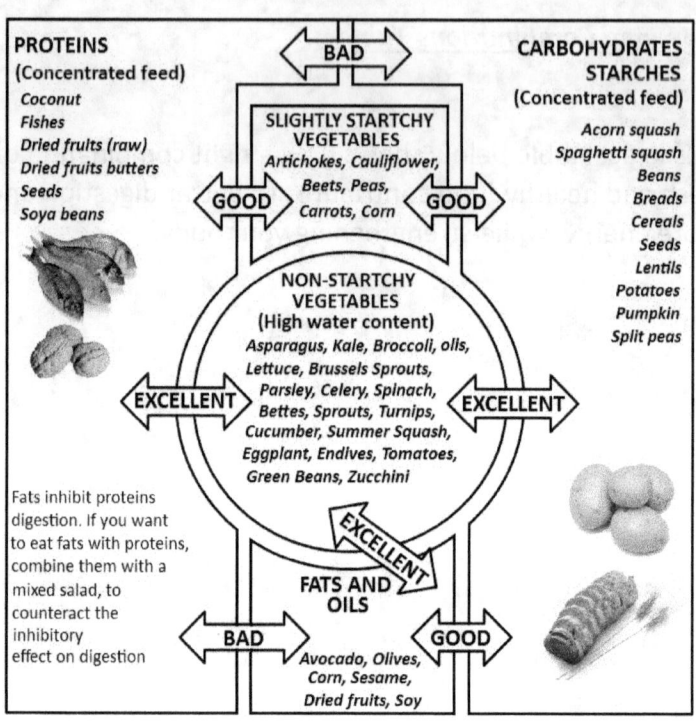

PROTEINS
(Concentrated feed)

Coconut
Fishes
Dried fruits (raw)
Dried fruits butters
Seeds
Soya beans

CARBOHYDRATES
STARCHES
(Concentrated feed)

Acorn squash
Spaghetti squash
Beans
Breads
Cereals
Seeds
Lentils
Potatoes
Pumpkin
Split peas

BAD

SLIGHTLY STARTCHY VEGETABLES
Artichokes, Cauliflower, Beets, Peas, Carrots, Corn

GOOD **GOOD**

NON-STARTCHY VEGETABLES
(High water content)
Asparagus, Kale, Broccoli, oils, Lettuce, Brussels Sprouts, Parsley, Celery, Spinach, Bettes, Sprouts, Turnips, Cucumber, Summer Squash, Eggplant, Endives, Tomatoes, Green Beans, Zucchini

EXCELLENT **EXCELLENT**

EXCELLENT

FATS AND OILS
Avocado, Olives, Corn, Sesame, Dried fruits, Soy

BAD **GOOD**

Fats inhibit proteins digestion. If you want to eat fats with proteins, combine them with a mixed salad, to counteract the inhibitory effect on digestion

FRUITS

SWEET	**MELON**	**SUB-ACID**	**ACIDIC**
Bananas	*Cantaloupe*	*Blackberries*	*Apple*
Dates	*Spanish Melon*	*Lemon*	*Cherries*
Dried fruits	*Watermelon*	*Orange*	*Peach*

1. Should always be eaten alone.
2. Melons should be eaten alone, or be mixed with acidic or sub-acid fruits.
3. Sweet fruits should be eaten after another fruit.

V.5- The Ideal Food Pyramid

The information conveyed by the traditional food pyramid made for decades by the USDA, is archaic and false.

The pyramid is focused on carbohydrates (for which it recommends 6 to 11 parts), and it also advises 2 to 3 portions of meat and dairy products per day. In other words: the ideal remedy to clog your body.

The latest version, even if it was improved, does not correct the problems of a diet based on the consumption of products of animal origin.

According to Anthony Robbins, the ideal food pyramid emphasizes, a predominantly vegetarian diet, including foods rich in water, such as fruits and vegetables. These cleansing foods should make up the bulk of your diet.

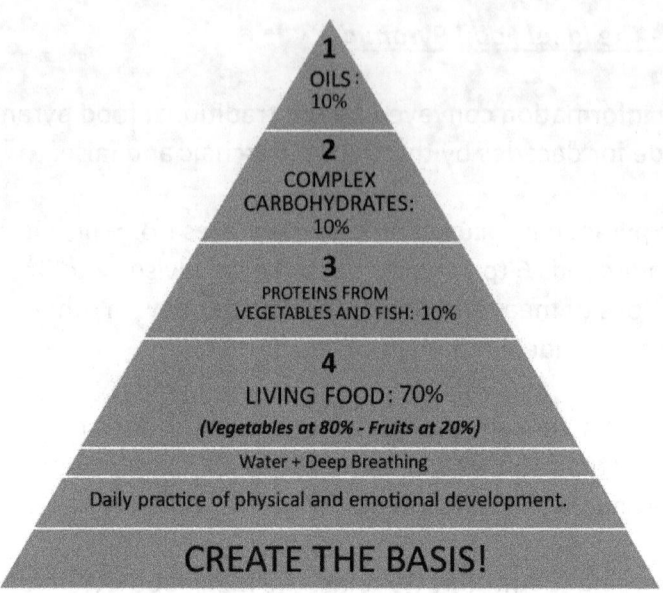

1 - OILS: 10%

2 - COMPLEX CARBOHYDRATES: 10%

3 - PROTEINS FROM VEGETABLES AND FISH: 10%

4 - LIVING FOOD: 70% (Vegetables at 80% - Fruits at 20%)

Water + Deep Breathing

Daily practice of physical and emotional development.

CREATE THE BASIS!

1- OILS: 10%

Olives, flax, Omega-3 and Omega-6, Udo's Oil, olive oil, avocados (do not heat cold pressed oils).

Good fats neutralize acids that attack the cell membrane and reduce saturated fats in the blood.

2- COMPLEX CARBOHYDRATES: 10%

Ideally, whole grains not stored, like basmati rice and jasmine rice, buckwheat, quinoa, millet, spelt, kamut, unleavened bread and noodles.

Indeed, cereals provide fibers that reduce toxicity.

3- PROTEINS FROM VEGETABLES AND FISH: 10%

Dried fruits, seeds and legumes, almonds, Brazil nuts, hazelnuts, lentils, nuts, pumpkin seeds, sunflower seeds.

Concerning fish, you will ideally want to choose deep water fish, such as salmon, tuna, halibut, albacore tuna, swordfish, snapper.

Proteins help in cell building.

4- LIVING FOOD: 70%

Vegetables at 80%:

Asparagus, broccoli, carrots, spinach, green pepper, celery, cucumber, lettuce, sprouts, wheat grass and fresh herbs.

Vegetables are an excellent source of vitamins, minerals, phytonutrients, antioxidants and fibers.

Fruits at 20%:

Ideally, fruits that are non acidic and not too sweet such as avocado, lemon, lime, tomato, grapefruit.

When the body is balanced, fruits are an excellent living food. To consume with moderation and only on an empty stomach.

V.6- Supplements Are Useful: 3 Levels To Optimize Your Life

Although we ideally try to get the quality nutrients we need from the food we eat, it is sometimes necessary to find somewhere else what could satisfy our body needs.

That's why we sometimes take supplements to make up our dietary deficiencies. These nutrients help us to a large extent like food: they help us to grow, keep our body and mind alert, help develop resistance to infection, and many more other things.

The Journal of the American Medical Association explains:

'There is evidence that sub-optimal levels of vitamins, well above those causing deficiency syndromes, are associated with an increased risk of chronic diseases, including cardiovascular disease, cancer and osteoporosis.'

In a clinical commentary, it is noted that 'a large part of the population' consumes a quantity of vitamins that is far from being optimal, which increases the risk of contracting diseases. And adds: 'It appears prudent for all adults to take vitamin supplements'

(Source: Journal of the American Medical Association Recent Articles June 2002)

****

MANY FOOD SUPPLEMENTS CAN BE ESSENTIAL FOR YOUR LIFE. THEY CAN BE TAKEN INTO ACCOUNT AT THREE LEVELS:

1. Creating the base: Stop poisoning and give your body what it needs.

7 Food supplements should be incorporated into your diet to create the daily basis.

2. Questioning yourself and changing: cleanse and detoxify your body.

The second family of supplements that we will consider is for your body cleansing. The goal here is to maintain the vitality of your body by eliminating the accumulated toxins due to your environment and lifestyle.

3. Celebrating and rewarding: Specific life experiences.

The third family of supplements to take depends on the specific short term goals and/or specific stages of your life.
****

1. Creating the base: Stop poisoning and give your body what it needs.

To create the basis and be healthy, you must stop poisoning and stop the bad habits that go against a life full of energy and vitality.

Remember, even if you do not feel bad, health is not the absence of disease, but the fact of living in top shape. Besides, to be balanced and create a solid basis, you must give your body the basic elements it needs in the form of food supplements.

7 ESSENTIAL NUTRIENTS TO COMPLETE YOUR DIET.

To enjoy an extraordinary health, it might be useful to include in your daily diet seven basic rituals:

1- Green vegetables
Green vegetables are alkalizing they cleanse and revitalize the body.

2- Digestive enzymes
If we fail to assimilate nutrients, we cannot take full advantage of what we eat. Digestive enzymes help us digest food more efficiently. They can also relieve symptoms associated with heartburn, irritable bowel syndrome or to other digestive disorders.

3- Oils

Balance your diet with essential fatty acids and products such as Udo's Perfect Blend Oil or Krill Oil. Udo's Perfect Blend and Twin Lab's Krill Essentials provide natural fatty acids with revitalizing and energizing power, and are recommended.

4- Acidophilus

In a society where there are now a plethora of anti-bacterial products, we do not always realize how much "good" bacteria are also eliminated by these products. Bacteria that are beneficial and necessary. Acidophilus replaces these helpful bacteria and helps us to achieve the right balance between beneficial bacteria and those who are new for our body.

5- Antioxidants

We rely on vitamins such as vitamins C and E to activate our defenses against free radicals that cause cellular aging. These supplements can also help prevent cancer, cardiovascular disease and other chronic diseases.

6. Multivitamins - "One per day"

Cooking and food processing often kill the nutrients they contain and force us to take food supplements. Multivitamins provide us with the essential vitamins and minerals we need, and that we cannot find in our diet.

7. Specific supplements

You may need additional nutraceuticals for example if you train with weights or if you are pregnant. If you suffer from arthritis, sore back or other ailments, there are many supplements that can relieve your symptoms.

2. Questioning yourself and changing: cleanse and detoxify your body.

With a good basis, you have enough resources to cope with difficulties and use them to grow and become stronger. The secret of health and a sustainable and vibrant energy consists in taking regularly the time to clean and detoxify your body.

In addition to providing a solid basis to end the poisoning, you need to cleanse your body of poisons you already ingested.

A diet and a hyper acidic lifestyle allow micro-organisms inside the bloodstream (yeasts, molds, fungi, etc.) to proliferate and to produce their own wastes (mycotoxins) that increase the toxicity of your body.

This is why it is ideal to make a detoxifying treatment at least once or twice a year to cleanse your body.

You can also purify and cleanse your body through food supplements available in natural or health food stores.

3. Celebrating and rewarding: Specific life experiences.

Finally, you must congratulate yourself, reward yourself and program yourself to win. In this journey towards the perfect health, it is important to celebrate this extraordinary feeling of having set new targets towards vitality.

Have you always wanted to climb a mountain, to finish a triathlon, to snowboard or beat any of your personal records?

When we reach this ultimate level of efficiency, it is important to celebrate it.
Depending on the situation, the goal and the expected result, it might be useful to take additional nutraceuticals. There are a variety of supplements that may be helpful to strengthen and improve the functioning of your body if you train with weights, you are pregnant, you have heart problems or if you have osteoarthritis, back pain or other ailments.

Many products are available in different brands, in natural or health food stores.

Prefer natural supplements extracted from real foods. Indeed, synthetic supplements are more difficult to absorb and to assimilate by the body. Select products that contain no binder or filler ingredients, because they can also adversely affect the process of digestion.

Remember that supplements are meant to be used in addition to fruits, vegetables and whole grains contained in your diet and do not replace them. Antioxidants, multivitamins and others, are here to strengthen even more the healthy diet you have set up to feed yourself optimally.

V.7- Ideal Menus Meal By Meal: Breakfast

IN THE MORNING, BREAK THE FAST.

Start the day with green vegetables and/or alkalizing foods juice. Upon awakening, you must detoxify your body, not clog it. For example, try a vegetable stock or some slightly sweetened fruit juices.

MONDAY	Steam broccoli with olive oil and lemon juice	Miso soup, spinach and green vegetables with lemon juice and lime seasoned with Udo's Choice Perfect Oil Blend
TUESDAY	Toast of bread with sprouted wheat avocado, tomato and seasoning (eg., Mrs. Dash®)	Vegetable juice (mixture of carrots, celery, parsley and wheat grass)
WEDNESDAY	Grilled Vegetable Bouillon (diced zucchini and yellow squash) green salad with crispy noodles and peas	Basmati rice with slices of avocado and tomato with lemon juice
THURSDAY	Tomato, cucumber and avocado salad with olive oil and lemon juice	Blend of fresh melon and / or grapefruit (after 30 days of healthy life and detoxification and only on an empty stomach)
FRIDAY	Sautéed broccoli in sesame oil, Bragg Liquid Aminos amino acids, Chinese five spices powder, sesame seeds	Basmati rice with broccoli and cauliflower, seasoned with olive oil and real salt and pepper
SATURDAY	Sautéed vegetables and potatoes mats with green peppers and onions	Vegetable juices (celery mixture, cucumber, parsley and spinach) and tomato, cucumber and avocado salad with olive oil and lemon
SUNDAY	Steam broccoli with olive oil and lemon juice, spices and sesame seeds	Miso soup and cucumber, tomato and avocado salad

AGAINST WRINKLES, TRY WHAT FOLLOWS...

Instead of using overpriced creams and treatments, see nutrition as a way to remove wrinkles.

Studies showed that consumption of whole grains, fruits, vegetables, legumes, and fatty acids Omega-3 can help the skin stay young and healthy.

Choose foods rich in lycopene, an antioxidant found in many red fruits and vegetables (especially watermelon and pink grapefruit); in beta-carotene, a form of vitamin A (it is found in red, orange and yellow foods, such as apricots, mangoes and sweet potatoes); and in vitamin B (found in yogurt, chickpeas, mushrooms and lentils).

V.8- Ideal Menus Meal By Meal: Lunch

IF YOU WANT TO EAT FOODS THAT WILL CLOG YOUR BODY, SUCH AS MEAT OR SUGAR, LUNCH IS THE RIGHT TIME TO DO IT.

You will give your body the ability to digest and detoxify through the remainder of the day.

MONDAY	Crepe (wrap) vegetables (germinated pepper tortilla, raw vegetables, dried tomatoes, almonds, etc.)	Grilled zucchini, peppers, cauliflower and broccoli on millet
TUESDAY	Tuna burger on a sprouted wheat bread with fresh tomato salad, lettuce and greens	Grilled eggplant on whole wheat focaccia with roasted peppers with pesto and tomato-spinach soup
WEDNESDAY	Warm spinach salad with falafel	Finely chopped salad (romaine lettuce finely chopped, tomatoes, cucumber, pine nuts, dried tomatoes, herbs, olive oil and basil)
THURSDAY	Grilled vegetables pancake with hummus and tabbouleh	Nicoise salad (tuna, potatoes with red skin, green beans, olives, romaine lettuce, lemon vinaigrette)
FRIDAY	Lentil soup with vegetables salad and crackers without yeast	Tortilla fish (halibut, vegetables, guacamole and tomato sauce)
SATURDAY	Burger of vegetables on a sprouted wheat bread with avocado, lettuce, tomato and sweet potato fries	Carrot/ginger soup with zucchini salad (zucchini, romaine lettuce and oak salad, radishes and onions, garlic dressing, linseed oil and salt)
SUNDAY	Vegetarian Chili and yellow pumpkin	Pancake with vegetables and hummus in a pita.

WHAT IF WE HAD FUN?

Some delicious and fun ideas for lunch to take away or for the snack break:

- Mini tortilla rolls with hummus and vegetables.

- Ready to eat bags with spinach salad, carrots, cucumbers and nuts with lemon.

- Cut celery to soak in a little almond butter jar.

V.9- Ideal Menus Meal By Meal: Diner

EAT SEVERAL HOURS BEFORE YOU GO TO BED.

Sleep should be a state of rest; your body should not have to work overtime at night to digest what you ate (which means agitated night for you). Do not eat cooked food late at night, prefer a light meal consisting of fresh and living food (easier to digest).

MONDAY	Grilled halibut with pesto sauce, asparagus, tomato, cucumber and avocado salad	Tofu and vegetables curry (peppers, carrots, broccoli, cauliflower, onions, garlic, etc.) with wild rice
TUESDAY	Grilled salmon, salad with asparagus and spinach, lemon tofu cheesecake	Cream of broccoli (soy milk) and rolled pancake with grilled vegetables
WEDNESDAY	Sautéed vegetables seasoned with Bragg Liquid Aminos, wild rice and miso soup	Vegetable fajitas with guacamole sauce, gazpacho and vegetable salad with clover sprouts, pine nuts, roasted peppers and olive oil
THURSDAY	Minestrone, spaghetti, tomato-basil sauce	Baked salmon, olive oil, rosemary, salt and pepper; sautéed spinach with garlic and green salad with olive oil and lemon
FRIDAY	Split pea soup and tortilla fish with lettuce, tomatoes, guacamole sauce (optional: soy sour cream)	Wonton soup (without eggs or mushrooms), Szechuan shrimps and peas, black bean sauce (without glutamates)
SATURDAY	Pizza without yeast, tomato sauce, grilled vegetables and rice mozzarella	Lentil soup, pita slices and salad of young mixed vegetables, flaxseeds, lentils sprouts, tomatoes, cucumber)
SUNDAY	Grilled tuna with herbs, vegetable medley, salad of young vegetables with flax seeds, lemon juice and olive oil	Rice or spelt pasta, pesto sauce, cabbage, carrots and pine nuts, toasted garlic and vegetable salad with tomatoes, cucumber, flax seeds, and avocado

TO TRY...

Add a little more to your water with a slice of lemon or mint.

These small living food touches will awaken your senses and help you detoxify your body.

VI- FIRST POISON: ELIMINATE OR SIGNIFICANTLY REDUCE INDUSTRIAL FATS

What is the problem of these industrial fats and why are they bad for you?

Butter, margarine, cheese, french fries, chips, cookies and other snacks are full of industrial fats.

The main fats in our diet are saturated fats, polyunsaturated, monounsaturated and trans fatty acids.

Americans consume an average of 35 to 40% of their calories in fats. Saturated fats, "trans" fats and dietary cholesterol raise the blood cholesterol level.

The bad news is that high blood cholesterol levels are a major risk for coronary heart disease, which can cause heart attack and also increases the risk of attack.

1- WHAT ARE INDUSTRIAL FATS OR TRANS FATTY ACIDS?

These are man-made fats or processed from liquid oil. When you hydrogenate a liquid vegetable oil and then you put it under pressure, it results in a more solid fat, like the one you can find in butter substitutes. The "trans" fats are also called hydrogenated fats.

2- WHY WORRYING OF PROCESSED FATTY ACIDS?

Clinical studies show that trans fatty acids or hydrogenated fats tend to increase the total level of cholesterol in the blood and of LDL cholesterol ("bad cholesterol"), while lowering HDL cholesterol ("good cholesterol"), when they are used instead of cis fatty acids (naturally produced) or instead of natural oils. Their consumption may increase the risk of heart disease.

According to the Nurses' Health Study, the largest survey on women and chronic diseases, "trans" fats double the risk of cardiovascular disease among women.

A recent study, on ten years, showed similar results: men who eat more "trans" fats have twice more chances to have a heart attack.

Industrial fats are also a danger for circulation and elimination, and they cause congestion and toxicity problems in the body.

3- ARE ALL THE FATS BAD?

No, all fats are not bad!

"Good fats" are an essential source of energy for the body. These "good" unsaturated fats contain essential fatty acids Omega-3 that help reduce the risk of cardiovascular disease and cancer. Some unsaturated oils are also used by the body for the formation of the cell wall and allow a proper neurological functioning.

The Committee of the American Heart Association Nutrition urges Americans who have been healthy for more than two years to limit their intake of saturated and "trans" fats: they recommend to get less than 7% of calories from saturated fats and less than 1% from processed fats.

In addition, the Food and Drug Administration (FDA) asked producers to show the "trans" fats level on food labels to help consumers avoid them more easily. The deadline for the application of this rule was the 1st of January 2006.

VI.1- How To Reduce Trans Acids In Your Food

- Use olive oil and garlic instead of butter.

- Limit industrial pastries and cakes (cookies, cakes, pies).

- Limit snacks to nibble and crisps.

- Avoid fried foods at the restaurant.

- Limit prepared dishes.

Industrial fats are fats that are destroyed during the baking process (at a temperature higher than 48 °C or 118.4°F), which makes them impossible to consume and toxic for the organism. This is how they can cause acidity and disease. There are industrial fats in butter, margarine, cheese, whole milk, meat, etc.

The dangers of bad fats (or industrial fats) are real: poor circulation (which leads to high blood pressure), difficult elimination, excessive congestion and toxicity of the body.

In addition, the body is no longer able to perform the same functions as with good fats (or non-industrial fats).

And above all: do not forget the essential fatty acids.

VI.2- Natural Fats, Not Processed, Serve Five Major Functions

1- They build the cell membrane.

2- They contribute to hormonal production.

3- They speed up metabolism and create energy.

4- They protect the body from acids and neutralize them.

5- They lubricate the body so that cells can move freely.

Non-industrial fats are the fats found in nature. The best examples are the fats in avocados, olive oil, almonds and flaxseed oil.

VII- SECOND POISON: ELIMINATE OR SIGNIFICANTLY REDUCE ANIMAL FLESH

We know that fats and oils are bad for us, and that coffee and other addictions are not that good.

But meat and dairy products are present in most Western diets (and more and more internationally), and it may be difficult to imagine life without a milkshake with strawberries, or a good steak in a cheeseburger.

The truth is that conventional ideas about nutrition kill us, bringing with them their train of heart disease, cancer, obesity, etc. We must open our minds to new ways of eating, and that means a predominantly vegetarian diet.

In "The Food Revolution: How Your Diet Can Help Save Your Life and Our World", John Robbins, an internationally recognized author, presents some statistics to help us understand the negative consequences of a predominantly carnivorous diet.

VII.1- Negative Consequences Of A Predominantly Carnivorous Diet

CARDIOVASCULAR DISEASE

- Risk of death from heart disease in vegetarians compared with non vegetarians: Half less.

- The level of blood cholesterol in vegetarians compared to non-vegetarians is 14% lower.

- Decrease of the risk of heart disease by reduction percentage of blood cholesterol: 3 to 4%.

- Incidence of hypertension among meat eaters compared to vegetarians: 13 times higher.

CANCER

- Impact on the risk of lung cancer for those who frequently eat green vegetables, oranges and yellows: reduction by 20 to 60%.

- The most common cancer in the US is the prostate cancer. Risk of developing a prostate cancer for men who consume a lot of cruciferous (broccoli, Brussels sprouts, cabbage, cauliflower, cabbage green cabbage curly, brown mustard and turnips): reduced by 41%.

- Risk of contracting colon cancer for women who eat red meat daily compared with those who eat red meat less than once per month: 250% higher.

VII.2- The China Study From Dr Campbell

Dr. T. Colin Campbell is at the forefront of nutrition research for more than 40 years. It is, inter alia:

- Winner of the Jacob Gould Shuman price and Professor Emeritus of Nutritional Biochemistry at Cornell University.

- Winner of the Research Prize in 1998, awarded by the American Institute for Cancer Research.

- He has given interventions in congressional committees and federal agencies; he participated in over 25 TV shows and documentaries; and has been the subject of numerous articles in USA Today or The New York Times.

- His research work has been funded by an amount equivalent to 74 year-scholarships and he is the author and co-author of over 350 scientific articles.

- He led the China Study (The China Study: Startling Implications for Diet, Weight Loss and Long-term Health), which is the most thorough study of health and nutrition ever conducted. Under his leadership, the current study began in 1983 in partnership with the Universities of Cornell and Oxford, and the Chinese Academy of Preventive Medicine.

After more than 40 years of research on the impact of nutrition on health, Dr. Campbell concluded that cancer, cardiovascular disease, diabetes and many of the diseases affecting our society can be prevented or treated via a diet consisting primarily of plants and complete feeds.

As part of his research funded by a grant of 27 years from the National Institute of Health (NIH), the American Cancer Society, and the American Institute for Cancer Research, Dr. Campbell made several specific findings on proteins:

- A low protein diet inhibits the initiation of cancer by aflatoxin, a mycotoxin found in peanuts and corn (aflatoxin is one of the most potent carcinogens ever discovered).

- After the initiation of cancer, a low protein diet blocks all subsequent development of cancer.

- Cancer is fed by casein, present at 87% in cow's milk.

- Even at high doses, "safe" plant proteins do not feed the cancer.

Proteins are essential components in a healthy body. They take the form of enzymes, hormones, structural tissues and transport the molecules that are necessary for life. Proteins are long chains of amino acids. When they "run out", they must be replaced by the foods we eat: When we digest food with proteins, the amino acids they contain are metabolized to create new proteins in the body.

It is said that food proteins are of different quality, depending on whether they provide more or less efficiently the amino acids we need to synthesize new tissue proteins. According to these measurements, high quality proteins come from human flesh, followed by animal flesh.

But a high efficiency in the synthesis of new proteins does not necessarily mean the best health possible.

Vegetable proteins of "inferior quality" allow a slow but steady synthesis of new proteins, and constitute the best proteins for the health.

All Campbell's findings lead to the same conclusion: those who consume the most foods from animal origin are infected with more chronic diseases. Small amounts of these foods already have harmful effects.

VII.3- Chicken: A Safe Alternative?

Contrary to popular beliefs, chicken is not a healthy alternative to red meat. Eating poultry is often much worse than eating beef.

The passage of a chicken from farm to fork is a painful process, during which the poisoning possibilities are numerous.

Before being extracted from their overcrowded cages, chickens are exposed to different levels of contamination. They are thrown into a hot water bath and sent to the feather removal machine.

At the end of the process, the chickens are immersed in a cooling bath, called "fecal soup", which is a reservoir of wastes and bacteria.

According to Gerald Kuester, a former microbiologist at the USDA:

"Modern slaughter technologies have created more than fifty points during the slaughter process where cross contamination can occur. At the end of the chain, the birds are as clean as if they had been dipped in the toilets."

TO THINK ABOUT...

If the quality of your health is not enough to discourage you from eating chicken, here are some disturbing facts about how chickens are slaughtered.

Did you know that four or more chickens are crammed in tiny farming cages, so they cannot stand up nor open their wings?

Or that the youngest one have their beak snatched without anesthesia to prevent them from hurting each other in these confined breeding conditions?

Or that modern breeding methods, the use of growth hormones and artificial lighting make many chickens grow faster than their bones, causing fractures and broken legs?

VII.4- Advices To Follow If You Choose To Continue To Eat Meat

1- Don't eat meat more than once a day!

2- Combine your portion of meat with lots of water-rich foods. Plan in the same meal a salad or steamed vegetables that will purify and not clog your body. Try to eat only cleansing foods during the rest of the day.

3- Eat meat at lunch time. This way, you give your body enough time to digest and you could still eat cleansing foods during the rest of the day.

4- Choose Meat that is:

     (A) Free-range
     (B) Kosher
     (C) guaranteed without antibiotics
     (D) Organic

5- Do not eat red meat and always choose the leanest cuts.

6- Go for seafood: it is an excellent choice for proteins, essential fatty acids and nutrition in general, as far as their origin is natural and clean.

TO THINK ABOUT...

If you like meat, you should know what produces the taste and texture of beef and chicken:

The taste comes from the uric acid, or urine, of the animal. Uric acid is extremely toxic and can cause arthritis pain.

Texture, soft and easy to chew, comes from putrefaction bacteria that tenderize the meat. These bacteria come from the colon, spread throughout the body of the animal that has been shot and soften the tissues so they can be consumed.

VIII- THIRD POISON: ELIMINATE OR SIGNIFICANTLY REDUCE DAIRY PRODUCTS

Cows do not drink cow's milk... Why should you drink some?

The medical profession and the media constantly encourage us to drink milk and eat dairy products "because it is good for us."

It could not be further from the truth...

VIII.1- The Myth Of Milk

Dairy products are fashionable and are the subject of numerous articles in the media. Many people are seduced by the advertising campaigns and white mustache of the stars in it, and say that this type of food is a 'plus' for health.

Many believe that milk and dairy products "are our friends for life" and help fight degenerative diseases, such as osteoporosis.

But what do you really know about this white liquid? The truth is that there are much better sources of calcium that these dairy products with a high level of proteins and fats.

Recent studies on the effects of dairy products proved that they widely contribute to osteoporosis, kidney problems and some cancers. In the study on the proteins of Dr. T. Colin Campbell, it appears that cancer is heavily supplied with casein, which represents 87% of the proteins in cow's milk.

In addition, women who have a diet rich in animal products excrete more calcium in their urine, and thus have a negative calcium balance, which represents a high risk for osteoporosis (source: *http://en.wikipedia.org/wiki/Osteoporosis*).

VIII.2- What Is Calcium And Why Do I Need It?

Calcium is a mineral that the body needs for many functions: development and maintenance of bones and teeth, blood clotting, nerve impulse transmission and regulation of heart rate. 99% of calcium in the human body is found in the bones and teeth. The remaining percent is in the blood and other tissues. The body gets the calcium it needs in two ways: by eating calcium rich foods and by the using the calcium stock located in the bones (source: Calcium and Milk: Sources Nutrition, Harvard School of Public Health, 2004.
http://www.hsph.harvard.edu/nutritionsource/calcium.html).

Animal proteins increase the acid burden in the body, i.e. of the degree of acidity of the blood and tissues. To neutralize the acidity, the body draws calcium in the bones and thus weakens them.

A recent report in the Journal of Pediatrics postulates that encouraging consumption of milk and milk products is not necessarily the best way to get the 400 milligrams of calcium that constitute the minimum intake.

VIII.3- What Is Osteoporosis?

Osteoporosis is a bone disease in which 1) the bone density decreases, 2) the internal spongy tissue resistance decreases, and 3) the surface of the bone becomes thinner, which increases the risk of fractures. Fractures of the spine, hip and wrist are typical.

The crushing of the vertebrae causes chronic pain and a characteristic deviation of the column, while fractures of long bones reduce the mobility and may require a surgical procedure. The hip fracture can cause permanent disability.

Ten million Americans suffer from osteoporosis and 34 million have osteopenia or decreased bone density, a disease that leads to osteoporosis and that is responsible for more than 2 million fractures each year. About 50% of women and 25% of men are likely to suffer from osteoporosis in their lifetime. (Source: Natural Osteoporosis Foundation - What is Osteoporosis 2005. *http://www.nof.org/osteoporosis/*).

VIII.4- What Can You Do To Prevent Osteoporosis?

Treatments exist, but there is no cure for osteoporosis, hence the need for prevention. Dr. Campbell made a series of recommendations to reduce the risk of osteoporosis: stay physically active, eat a variety of plant foods, avoid animal foods (including dairy) and limit your salt intake to a minimum.

Other recommendations to prevent osteoporosis (source: National Osteoporosis Foundation NOF's Five Steps to Bone Health and Osteoporosis Prevention of 2002. *http://nof.org/prevention/*):

a) Exercise regularly with weights.

b) Consume the daily recommended doses of calcium and vitamin D.

c) Do not abuse caffeine, alcohol and tobacco.

Also, if you want healthy bones:

- Do not smoke, do not start

- Avoid alcohol abuse

- Limit caffeine

- Make more exercise!

VIII.5- Les Conséquences Of Dairy Products Consumption

Dairy products harm your body in several ways:

1- CANCER

Breast milk, human or animal, carries hundreds of chemicals, including a hormone, the IGF-1 (Insulin-like Growth Factor). Milk consumption increases the circulation of this hormone in the body and high IGF-1 levels are associated with prostate cancer, colorectal cancer, premenopausal breast cancer and lung cancer.

In nine separate studies, the recurring dietary factor in cases of prostate cancer was high consumption of milk and dairy products. In the most important of these studies, the Health Professionals Follow-Up Study, men who drank at least two glasses of milk per day had almost twice more risk of developing advanced prostate cancer than those who did not drink milk at all (source: "Food Can Trigger an Asthma Attack: Up to 10% of Cases," Bykownski, Mike, Family Practice News, (1997); 60.).

2- MUCUS PRODUCTION

Milk and dairy products tend to generate an excess of mucus in the intestines, sinuses and lungs. In the intestine, this excessive mucus hardens and form, on the inner wall, a substantially impermeable layer to nutrients. Nutrients absorption is thus affected, which leads to chronic fatigue. Milk consumption is also a factor that contributes to the runny nose and to an excess of mucus in the throat.

3- ALLERGIES

Very few adults properly metabolize the protein contained in cow's milk. Nearly 10% of asthma cases could be related to food allergies. Food allergy is the leading cause of anaphylaxis outside the hospital, and milk contributes to a large part of the reactions.

4- MORE

Studies showed that dairy products can also be involved in many other health problems: irritable bowel syndrome, malabsorption of nutrients, obesity and deficiencies of minerals and amino acids.

VIII.6- Don't Children Need Milk To Grow Well And Have Strong Bones?

Do children who consume milk have stronger bones? The mighty dairy industry would like us to believe it!

In a press release, Dairy Management, Inc. (American organization dedicated to promoting the sale of American-made dairy products) presented its objectives:

Sell to young children and their mothers, use schools to reach young consumers, conduct and produce research favorable to the industry. In 2002, the website of the organization offered more than 70,000 lesson plans to educators.

Campbell observed:

"The dairy industry really teaches its own version of nutrition to younger generations."

An article published recently in the Journal of Pediatrics by researchers at the 'Medical Committee for Responsible Medicine' of Washington, reviews the results of 37 studies on the impact of calcium consumption on bone strength in children of more than 7 years, and notes that 27 of these studies do not endorse the idea that we need to drink more milk to increase the calcium level (source: Amy Joy Lanou, PhD, Susan E. Berkow, PhD CN et Neal D. Barnard, MD. "Calcium, Dairy Products and Bone Health in Children and Young Adults: A Reevaluation.").

This is the physical activity of young people that is considered to be the main reason of bones growth and development.

THINK ABOUT IT...

"Cow milk contains hormones which are secreted by the pituitary gland of the animal."

This statement, made several years ago by Dr. Michael Rabbens, Phoenixville Pennsylvania, is confirmed by many researchers.

"These are potent growth hormones, a calf that weighs 88 pounds at birth reaches 990 pounds at its physical maturity, two years later. By comparison, a baby weighs between 5.95 and 7 lb at birth, and between 99 and 198 pounds when he reaches its physical maturity 21 years later."

VIII.7- Other Sources Of Calcium

There are now on the market many delicious alternatives; so you do not have to permanently abandon your favorite foods to maintain a good nutritional balance: there is soy milk, rice milk, rice, yogurt or soy, or sesame seed milk.

In absolute terms, dairy products contain as much calcium as calcium-rich plants. However, when one takes into account absorption, the amount of plant food necessary to obtain a quantity of absorbable calcium that is equivalent to that of dairy products, is modest.

For example, to get the same amount of absorbable calcium provided by a cup of cow's milk, you can choose between a cup of soy milk, a cup of kale or turnip greens, two packages of quick cooking oatmeal, two-thirds of a cup of tofu, or a cup and a half of broccoli.

IX- FOURTH POISON: ELIMINATE OR SIGNIFICANTLY REDUCE ACIDIC ADDICTIONS

A diet that promotes the over-acidification of the blood and tissues creates a breeding ground for viruses, bacteria and fungi, great destroyers of cells and tissues in the human body.

Think of it in these terms: a refrigerator must remain cold to protect the food from bacteria, fungi and mold.

If the environment created by the refrigerator is threatened and if the refrigerator starts to warm up, the food contained in it will develop bacteria that will turn into yeasts and molds. The food will then degrade and be spoiled.

It happens exactly the same in your body when you eat too much of acidifying foods. This is how all infectious and degenerative diseases start.

WHAT IS THE SOLUTION?

To reduce and eliminate acidic substances, you need a diet consisting of living alkaline foods: Dark green and yellow vegetables, soybeans, sprouted oil seeds, seeds, grains and essential fatty acids. Such a diet will reduce the over-acidification of the blood and tissues by its abundance of basis and alkaline salts.

SAY **NO** TO ACIDIC ADDICTIONS:		
1- CAFFEINE	5- "WHITE" PRODUCTS	
2- SUGAR	6- VINEGAR	
3- NICOTINE	7- PHARMACEUTICALS	
4- ALCOHOL		

IX.1- *Caffeine*

Caffeine is a toxic alkaloid and is the active ingredient of all the beverages we seem not to be able to do without, such as coffee, tea, cocoa and sodas. In the global exchanges in dollars, coffee is the second commodity after oil. Every year, more than 500 billion of cups of coffee are drunk in the World!

YOU KILL YOURSELF WITH CAFFEINE

Caffeine can jeopardize health and vitality by weakening the body.

- Caffeine stimulates the adrenal glands to produce adrenaline and cortisone, hormones that the body uses to raise the heart rate, speed up breathing and blood pressure. The adrenal glands become exhausted and can no longer meet the high solicitations, making the body more vulnerable to face the various health threats.

- It can seriously affect the cardiovascular system (hypertension, increased cholesterol, or arrhythmia and palpitations among the most sensitive people), digestive system (stomach pain, ulcers, diarrhea, malabsorption of nutrients) and energy expenditure of the body.

- Possible links between caffeine and disease: bladder cancer in men, breast cancer in women, and birth defects (in case of consumption during pregnancy).

- Caffeine can also have other consequences: nervousness, anxiety, irritability, muscle tremors, insomnia, chronic fatigue and headaches.

TO THINK ABOUT...

When the level of glucose in the body increases, the pancreas responds by releasing an excessive amount of insulin in the body. Sugar is quickly burnt, producing an energy peak (top).

The level of sugar in the blood then drops below the normal level, which is accompanied by unpleasant symptoms (down) such as headaches, excessive hunger, tremors, fatigue and like any drug, an incomprehensible desire to consume more.

In addition, a high insulin level inhibits the release of growth hormones, which depresses the immune system. It causes a feeling of "hunger" and increases fats storage.

IX.2- Sugar

Processed or refined sugar should be avoided. It is highly acidic and causes a rapid rise in glucose level in blood.

Glucose is the first substance metabolized by yeast, bacteria, molds and fungi in the body. This is what creates a hyper-acidic environment, where disease and its symptoms can develop. Sugar is an addictive substance that causes diabetes, obesity, thrombosis, dental caries and periodontal disease, varicose veins, stomach problems and, indirectly, mental disorders.

The primary source of sugar in our diet? Sodas.

The consumption of these soft drinks per capita increased by 500% since the fifties, the United States consume each day more than 50 million of Cokes!

According to the National Association of Refreshing drinks, a normal soda of 12 fl oz contains the equivalent of 10 teaspoons of sugar and 150 calories.

This amount of sugar can stop nearly 33% of the immune system (thirty spoons of sugar are sufficient to immobilize it an entire day).

TRUTH: SUGAR = ACID = GLUE IN YOUR BODY

IX.3- Nicotine

The negative effects of nicotine abuse are well known: risk of cardiovascular disease, lung cancer, stroke, emphysema and hypertension.

Nicotine also has adverse effects on memory: L. Binet has shown that when nicotine is put into the water of an aquarium, fishes lose memory.

In the United States, tobacco is responsible for nearly 1 in 5 deaths, equivalent to 443 000 deaths each year from 2000 to 2004. (Source: Cancer Facts and Figures 2010).

In summary, smoking puts you at risk and endangers people around you.

IX.4- Alcohol

According to Dr. Melvin H. Knisely of the Medical Faculty of South Carolina in Charleston, *"every time a person drinks a glass of alcohol, it causes irreversible damages to his brain, killing thousands of cells."*

IX.5- "White Food"

Take the habit to avoid all the "white" food: wheat-based products, breads, rice, sugar and potatoes. Indeed, such kind of food are carbohydrates with a high glycemic index: their consumption will cause an insulin spike.

In addition, stored cereals (wheat, rice, barley) begin to ferment after 90 days in most cases and are rapidly filled with mycotoxins. This is a natural process that is regulated but inevitable. (Note: corn and peanuts can easily be contaminated with fungi)

IX.6- Vinegar

Vinegar is the result of decomposition, it contains acetic acid which affects the liver, a bit like alcohol. Vinegar thickens the blood, which affects the functioning of arteries and heart. It also interferes with the digestion of starch.

IX.7- Pharmaceuticals

The dangers of drugs are obvious, but the potential dangers of pharmaceutical drugs with a medical prescription are on less known.

Millions of dollars are spent each year to praise the positive effects of these so-called miraculous drugs. The public is increasingly aware of the risks, since the popular pharmaceutical drugs had to be instantly removed due to several disasters (such as Vioxx, after it was discovered that it doubled the risk of heart attack for the user).

Pharmaceuticals with medical prescription can also have side effects, but over-the-counter medications should not be considered 100% safe.

The Aleve (also known as Naproxen) made newspapers headlines when it was linked to an increase of 50% of heart attacks. Common painkillers can irritate the stomach or cause bleeding, and some drugs against allergies have side effects and cause cardiac arrhythmia. (Source: Health and Fitness, April 17, 2005).

X- YOUR DETOX ACTION PLAN FOR A LIFE OF PURE ENERGY, SHAPE AND HEALTH

Now that you have all the necessary tools to detoxify yourself, to eat well and to create a life of pure energy, shape and health, how are you going to use them?

What principles are you going to adopt in your daily routine to enjoy the quality of life you have always dreamed of?

Here is an action plan specially designed to integrate all you learned here into your daily life, right today.

1- THE POWER OF WATER AND LIVING FOODS

1- Drink daily as many sips of water as half of your weight in pounds. (If you weigh 200 pounds, you should drink 100 sips of water every day).

2- Find a pure source:

   a) Water Filter Reverse Osmosis.

   b) Penta-Hydrate (www.pentawater.com) 2 to 3 times a day for maximum absorption.

3- Eat water rich food: at least 70% of your diet.

2- THE POWER OF ESSENTIAL OILS

Add to your diet the essential fatty acids your body needs (Omega-3, Omega-6), using the way you prefer among these ones:

1- Eat foods containing natural fats that are not processed: avocados, almonds, hazelnuts, pumpkin or sunflower seeds, flax oil, olive oil and fish.

2- Twin Lab's Krill Oil 300 mg/day.

3- Udo's Choice Oil Blend: 1 tablespoon per 55 pounds of body weight and per day.

3- THE POWER OF ALKALINITY: GO GREEN!

1- Consume 70 to 80% of living foods and alkali creators (green vegetables, almonds, avocados, lemons, etc.)

2- Avoid foods creators of acid and without life: animal meats, dairy products, refined white foods, sugar, caffeine, etc.

3. Supplement your diet with 'greens' of quality.

4. Test your pH.

5- Make it SIMPLE: Add fresh lemon to your water every day!

4- THE POWER OF OPTIMAL NUTRITION

1 Follow the five rules of healthy eating:

    1) Drink water before eating, not during.
    2) Combine your food (don't eat fruits on an empty stomach and eat green vegetables or a salad with proteins or carbohydrates; do not mix fats and proteins).
    3) Eat relax.
    4) Do not overeat (eat less to live longer, and thus to eat more!).
    5) Eat organic (no pesticides, antibiotics, growth hormones).

2. Beware of the 'Flash Sugar Effect': keep your blood sugar below 55.

3- Create your Ideal Food Pyramid: 70% of living food, 10% of vegetable proteins or quality fish, 10% of carbohydrates and 10% of quality oils.

4- In addition!

    1) Create the basis: Follow a daily diet with the 7 Vital Nutrients to build the foundation of health.
    2) Challenge and Evolution: Practice periodic cleaning of your internal organs and your body.
    3) Celebration and Award: Take nutritional supplements if necessary and thus maximize your results!

5- FIRST POISON: ELIMINATE OR SIGNIFICANTLY REDUCE INDUSTRIAL FATS

1- Eliminate or greatly reduce your consumption of industrial/hydrogenated fats.

2. Keep your daily fats intake below 25% (in other words: less than 25% of the calories you eat every day must be fats).

6- SECOND POISON: ELIMINATE OR SIGNIFICANTLY REDUCE ANIMAL FLESH

1- Eliminate or greatly reduce your consumption of animal flesh.

2- Your total proteins intake should not exceed 5 to 6% per day and shall be of plant origin, because they are more efficient and contain more antioxidants, fibers and minerals.

3- Try to meet the challenge of eliminating all animal flesh for at least 10 days. If after ten days you feel that you have to start eating animal flesh again, do not do it more than once a day and do it with green vegetables or a salad, at lunch time, kosher, organic and antibiotic-free.

7- THIRD POISON: ELIMINATE OR SIGNIFICANTLY REDUCE DAIRY PRODUCTS

1- Eliminate or greatly reduce your consumption of cow's milk-based products.

2- Your calcium intake should not exceed 400 milligrams per day and its origin must be vegetal. Cow's milk draws calcium from bones.

3- Try alternatives (in moderation) such as rice milk, soy or almonds for texture or taste.

8- FOURTH POISON: ELIMINATE OR SIGNIFICANTLY REDUCE ACIDIC ADDICTIONS

1- Eliminate or greatly reduce your intake of acids.

2. Use common sense! Say no to the following addictions: caffeine, sugar, 'white products', vinegar, alcohol, nicotine and pharmaceuticals. Think about the consequences and break the pattern.

3- Alkalize yourself! If you consume at least 70 to 80% of alkaline food and that give life, your body will naturally decrease its addiction to acids.

XI- MORE BOOKS FROM THE SAME AUTHOR

HOW TO CONCENTRATE LIKE EINSTEIN:
THE LAZY STUDENT'S WAY TO INSTANTLY IMPROVE MEMORY & GRADES
WITH THE DOCTOR VITTOZ SECRET CONCENTRATION TECHNIQUE

Concentrate now on what you want as long as you want by learning the never before revealed concentration technique used by Einstein.

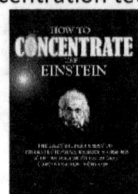

RESCUE ACUPRESSURE:
INSTANTLY SUPPRESS STRESS, HEADACHES, MEMORY LAPSES IN
DESPERATE SITUATIONS LIKE DURING AN EXAM

Relieve pain and discomfort immediately when you need it and do not let them make you fail an exam, a job interview or any important moment of your life. 100% practical, very clear and simple, this book is definitely the best investment you can do for your health and success.

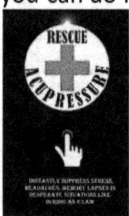

www.ingramcontent.com/pod-product-compliance
Lightning Source LLC
Chambersburg PA
CBHW072208280526
45788CB00002B/927